Contents

Gastritis is the main name used for any condition that involves inflammation of the stomach lining. Gastritis can be either acute (happens all of a sudden) or chronic (happens over time). There are different types of gastritis that are caused by different factors.

For most people, gastritis is minor and will go away quickly after treatment. There are some forms of gastritis that can produce ulcers or cause a higher risk for cancer.

Your diet is important for your digestive and overall health. What you put in your stomach can make a difference in the health of your digestive system. For instance, some forms of gastritis are caused by drinking alcohol too often or too much at one time. Avoiding some foods and beverages and eating others can help manage the condition.

What to Eat on A Gastritis Diet

There are some foods that may help manage your gastritis and lessen the symptoms. These include:

- High-fiber foods such as apples, oatmeal, broccoli, carrots, and beans

- Low-fat foods such as fish, chicken, and turkey breast

- Foods with low acidity, or are more alkaline, like vegetables

- Drinks that are not carbonated

- Drinks without caffeine

- Probiotics such as kombucha, yogurt, kimchi, and sauerkraut

Some studies show that probiotics may help with Helicobacter pylori (H. pylori). H. pylori is bacteria that causes an infection in the digestive system which can lead to gastritis or stomach ulcers.

1. Jacket Potatoes with Home-baked Beans

Prep: 10 Mins

Cook: 1 Hr, 30 Mins

Serves: 4

Ingredients

- 4 baking potatoes
- 1 tbsp sunflower oil
- 1 carrot, diced
- 1 celerystalk, diced
- 400g can haricot beans, drained
- 2 tomatoes, chopped
- 1 tsp paprika
    - choose sweet or hot depending on taste
- 1 tsp Worcestershire sauce
- 2 tbsp chopped chives, to serve

Directions

1. Heat oven to 200C/180C fan/gas 6. Scrub the potatoes and dry well, then prick in several places with a fork. Bake directly on the oven shelf for 1-1½ hrs, until they feel soft when squeezed.

2. After 30 mins, heat the oil in a pan and gently cook the carrot and celery for 10 mins until softened. Add the beans, tomatoes and paprika and cook gently for a further 5 mins until the tomatoes are softened and pulpy. Stir in 100ml water and the Worcestershire sauce, cook for a further 5 mins then cover and keep warm.

3. Split open the potatoes and spoon in the beans. Scatter with chives and serve.

2. Mustardy Beetroot & Lentil Salad

Prep: 5 Mins

Cook: 20 Mins

Serves: 5 – 6

Ingredients

- 200g puy lentils (or use 2 x 250g packs pre-cooked lentils)
- 1 tbsp wholegrain mustard (or gluten-free alternative)
- 1½ tbsp extra virgin olive oil
- 300g pack cooked beetroot (not in vinegar), sliced
- large handful tarragon, roughly chopped

Directions

1. If not using pre-cooked lentils, cook the lentils following pack instructions, drain and leave to cool. Meanwhile, combine the mustard, oil and some seasoning to make a dressing.
2. Tip the lentils into a bowl, pour over the dressing and mix well. Stir through the beetroot, tarragon and some seasoning, then serve.

3. Kale Tabbouleh

Prep: 15 Mins

Cook: 15 Mins

Serves: 6

Ingredients

- 100g bulgur wheat
- 100g kale
- large bunch mint, roughly chopped
- bunch spring onion, sliced
- ½ cucumber, diced
- 4 tomatoes, deseeded and chopped
- pinch of ground cinnamon
- pinch of ground allspice
- 6 tbsp olive oil
- juice and zest ½ lemon
- 100g feta cheese, crumbled
- 4 Baby Gem lettuces, leaves separated, to serve

Directions

1. Tip the bulgur wheat into a heatproof bowl and just cover with boiling water, then cover with cling film and set aside for 10-15 mins or until tender. Put the kale in a food processor and pulse to finely chop.

2. Stir the kale, mint, spring onions, cucumber and tomatoes through the bulgur wheat. Season with the cinnamon and allspice, then dress with the olive oil and lemon juice to taste. Scatter over the lemon zest and feta. To serve, let everyone scoop the salad onto leaves of Baby Gem lettuce.

4. Cranberry Chicken Salad

Prep: 15 Mins

Cook: 10 Mins

Serves: 4

Ingredients

- 2 skinless chicken breasts
- 4 tsp olive oil
- 2 red onions, thinly sliced

- 200g mixed leaves
- ½ cucumber, deseeded and sliced
- 25g dried cranberries
- 85g/3oz cranberry sauce
- juice 1 lime

Directions

1. Slice each chicken breast in half horizontally to give 4 thin breasts, then rub with half the oil and season. Heat a non-stick frying pan and fry the chicken for 3 mins on each side until cooked through. Set aside on a plate.

2. Heat the remaining oil in the pan and fry the onions for 5 mins. Slice the chicken, collecting any juices, and layer up with the onions, leaves, cucumber and dried cranberries. Mix the cranberry sauce, lime juice, 2 tbsp water and any chicken resting juices, and drizzle over the salad.

5. Spicy Bean Tostadas with Pickled Onions & Radish Salad

Prep: 15 Mins

Cook: 12 Mins

Serves: 4

Ingredients

- 2 red onions, 1 thinly sliced, 1 finely chopped
- 2 limes, juice of 1 and 1 cut into wedges
- 1½ tbsp sunflower oil
- 2 garlic cloves, finely chopped
- 2 tsp ground cumin
- 1 tbsp tomato purée
- 1 tbsp chipotle paste
- 400g can kidney bean, drained and rinsed
- 4 corn tortillas
- 140g radish thinly sliced
- large handful coriander, roughly chopped

Directions

1. Heat oven to 220C/200C fan/gas 7. Put the sliced onion, lime juice and seasoning in a bowl, and set aside.

2. Heat 1 tbsp of the oil in a pan and fry the chopped onion and garlic until tender. Stir in the cumin and fry for 1 min more. Add the tomato purée, chipotle paste and beans, stir, then tip in half a can of water. Simmer for 5 mins, season, then roughly mash to a purée. (You can cook for a few mins more if it is a bit runny, or add a few splashes of water to thin.)

3. Meanwhile, brush the tortillas with the remaining oil and place on a baking sheet. Bake for 8 mins until crisp. Spread the tortillas with the bean mixture. Mix the radishes and coriander with the pickled onions, then spoon on top. Serve with lime wedges.

6. Griddled Vegetable & Feta Tart

Prep: 10 Mins

Cook: 40 Mins

Serves: 4

Ingredients

- 2 tbsp olive oil
- 1 aubergine, sliced
- 2 courgettes, sliced
- 2 red onions, cut into chunky wedges
- 3 large sheets filo pastry
- 10-12 cherry tomatoes, halved
- drizzle of balsamic vinegar
- 85g feta cheese, crumbled
- 1 tsp dried oregano
- large bag mixed salad leaves and low-fat dressing, to serve

Directions

1. Heat oven to 220C/200C fan/gas 7. Pop 33 x 23cm baking tray in the oven to heat up. Brush a griddle

pan with about 1 tsp of the oil and griddle the aubergines until nicely charred, then remove. Repeat with the courgettes and onions, using a little more oil if you need to.

2. Remove the tray from the oven and brush with a little oil. Brush a large sheet of filo with oil, top with another sheet, add a little more oil and repeat with the final sheet. Transfer the pastry to the hot tray, pushing it into the edges a little.

3. Arrange the griddled veg on top, then season. Add the tomatoes, cut-side up, then drizzle on the vinegar and any remaining oil. Crumble on the feta and sprinkle with oregano. Cook for about 20 mins until crispy and golden. Serve with the dressed mixed salad leaves.

7. Chunky Mediterranean Tomato Soup

Prep: 10 Mins

Cook: 25 Mins

Serves: 4

Ingredients

- 400g frozen grilled vegetable mix (peppers, aubergine, onion, courgettes)
- 2 tbsp chopped garlic
- handful basil leaves
- 400g can chopped tomato
- 1 reduced-salt vegetable stock cube
- 50g ricotta per person, beaten with snipped chives and basil, spread on a slice of rye bread

Directions

1. Heat a large non-stick pan, tip in half the vegetables and the garlic, and cook, stirring, over a high heat until they start to soften – about 5 mins. Tip in the basil, tomatoes, stock cube and 2 cans of water, then blitz with a hand blender to get the mixture as smooth as you can.

2. Add the remaining frozen veg, cover the pan and cook for 15-20 mins more until the veg is tender. Ladle into bowls. Serve with the herby ricotta on rye bread.

8. Spinach & Pepper Frittata

Prep: 10 Mins

Cook: 40 Mins

Serves: 4

Ingredients

- 5 large eggs
- 300g tub low-fat natural cottage cheese
- 1 garlic clove, finely chopped
- 15g finely grated parmesan (or vegetarian alternative)
- 225g frozen leaf spinach, thawed, squeezed and finely chopped
- 2 roasted red peppers (not in oil), torn into strips
- generous grating of nutmeg
- 100g whole cherry tomato

Directions

1. Heat oven to 190C/170C fan/gas 5. Line a 20cm sandwich tin with a single sheet of baking parchment if your tin has a loose bottom.

2. Beat the eggs in a large bowl with the cottage cheese, garlic, half the Parmesan, the spinach, peppers, nutmeg and some black pepper. Tip into the tin, top with the tomatoes and sprinkle with the remaining Parmesan. Bake for 40 mins until set all the way through and starting to puff up. Cut into wedges and serve hot or cold. Will keep for 3-4 days in the fridge.

9. Chunky Butternut Mulligatawny

Prep: 25 Mins

Cook: 40 Mins

Serves: 6

Ingredients

- 2 tbsp olive or rapeseed oil
- 2 onions, finely chopped
- 2 dessert apples, peeled and finely chopped
- 3 celerysticks, finely chopped
- ½ small butternut squash, peeled, seeds removed, chopped into small pieces
- 2-3 heaped tbsp gluten-free curry powder (depending on how spicy you like it)
- 1 tbsp ground cinnamon
- 1 tbsp nigella seeds (also called black onion or kalonji seeds)
- 2 x 400g cans chopped tomatoes
- 1½ l gluten-free chicken or vegetable stock
- 140g basmati rice
- small pack parsley, chopped

- 3 tbsp mango chutney, plus a little to serve, if you like(optional)
- natural yogurt, to serve

Directions

1. Heat the oil in your largest saucepan. Add the onions, apples and celery with a pinch of salt. Cook for 10 mins, stirring now and then, until softened. Add the butternut squash, curry powder, cinnamon, nigella seeds and a grind of black pepper. Cook for 2 mins more, then stir in the tomatoes and stock. Cover with a lid and simmer for 15 mins.
2. By now the vegetables should be tender but not mushy. Stir in the rice, pop the lid back on and simmer for another 12 mins until the rice is cooked through. Taste and add more seasoning if needed. Stir through the parsley and mango chutney, then serve in bowls with yogurt and extra mango chutney on top, if you like.

10. Moroccan chickpea soup

Prep: 5 Mins

Cook: 20 Mins

Serves 4

Ingredients

- 1 tbsp olive oil
- 1 medium onion, chopped
- 2 celery sticks, chopped
- 2 tsp ground cumin
- 600ml hot vegetable stock
- 400g can chopped plum tomatoes with garlic
- 400g can chickpeas, rinsed and drained
- 100g frozen broad beans
- zest and juice ½ lemon
- large handful coriander or parsley and flatbread, to serve

Directions

1. Heat the oil in a large saucepan, then fry the onion and celery gently for 10 mins until softened,

stirring frequently. Tip in the cumin and fry for another min.

2. Turn up the heat, then add the stock, tomatoes and chickpeas, plus a good grind of black pepper. Simmer for 8 mins. Throw in broad beans and lemon juice, cook for a further 2 mins. Season to taste, then top with a sprinkling of lemon zest and chopped herbs. Serve with flatbread.

11. Chicken Zucchini Stir Fry

Prep Time: 15 Mins

Cook Time: 5 Mins

Total Time: 20 Mins

Yield: 4

Ingredients

- 1/4 cup low sodium soy sauce or use gf soy sauce*
- 1 cup chicken broth*
- 1 tablespoon cornstarch
- 2 tablespoons mirin
- 1 tablespoon sugar
- 2 teaspoons sesame oil
- 1 tablespoon canola oil divided
- 1 tablespoon minced garlic
- 1 tablespoon minced ginger
- 1 pound chicken breast, sliced very thinly
- 2 cups zucchini, cut 1/4 inch thick half moons (from 1 large zucchini)
- sesame seeds and scallion for garnish, if desired

Directions

1. In a large bowl add the soy sauce, chicken broth, cornstarch, mirin, sugar, and sesame oil and whisk until everything is completely dissolved.

2. In a large skillet add one teaspoon canola oil on medium high heat and cook half the chicken until just cooked through, about 2-3 minutes on each side. Set aside on a plate.

3. Repeat with the second half of the chicken and an additional teaspoon of oil. Remove the chicken to the plate.

4. Add in the remaining 1 teaspoon oil, garlic and ginger and cook for 30-45 seconds until very fragrant but not browned.

5. Stir the garlic and ginger well and add in the sauce, whisking well. Cook the sauce 1 minute, then add in the zucchini and cook for 2 minutes more, until thickened and the zucchini is tender crisp. Remove from heat, add in the chicken and stir well to coat. Garnish with sesame seeds and scallions if desired.

12. Garlicky Kale and White Bean Stew

Serves: 3-4

Preparation: 2min

Cooking: 15min

Ingredients

- 2 tspcoconut oil or ghee
- 2medium onions, sliced
- sea salt
- pinch chilli flakes
- 5bay leaves
- 1 tspsmoked paprika
- 6cloves garlic, sliced
- cracked black pepper
- 2-2 ½ cupscooked white beans (haricot, butter and/or cannelini)
- 2 cupspacked shredded kale leaves
- 2 cupsvegetable broth
- 1can (400 g) organic whole tomatoes
- cold-pressed olive oil to garnish

Directions

1. Heat oil in a large stockpot on medium heat. Add onions to the pot with a couple pinches sea salt, chilli, bay leaves and paprika. Cook for a few minutes until the onions have softened, then add garlic. If it looks dry, add a little juice from the tinned tomatoes.

2. Add all other ingredients, bring to a boil, season to taste, and serve in bowls with a drizzle of olive oil (since everything is cooked, you don't need to heat it long). If you are going to let it simmer for a while, add the kale about 5 minutes before serving so that it retains more of its nutritional value.

13. Kale Stir Fry with Crispy Curried Tofu

Prep Time: 10 Mins

Cook Time: 15 Mins

Servings: 2 People

Ingredients

- Crispy Curried Tofu
- 1 block (200g) Firm Tofu
- 1.5 tsp Curry Powder
- 1 tbsp Soy Sauce
- 1/4 Red Cabbage

Stir Fry

- 3-4 Large Kale Leaves
- 1 Carrot
- 1 clove garlic
- 1 inch piece Fresh Ginger
- 2 tbsp Soy Sauce
- 2 portions Wholewheat Noodles

Directions

1. Cut the tofu into 1 inch cubes. Mix together the curry powder and 1 tbsp soy sauce to make a paste. Add the tofu cubes and gently toss them so they are all coated with the sauce. Set aside while you prepare the other ingredients.
2. Boil the noodles according to the packet. While they are cooking, get on with the rest of the stir fry.
3. Slice the carrot very finely (or spiralize if you have one), and mince the ginger and garlic. Slice the cabbage and kale into thin strips.
4. Prep 2 frying pans with a little oil and heat on high.
5. To the first frying pan, add the tofu, and cook until golden brown on all sides, turning the pieces frequently. At the same time, cook the stir fry in the other frying pan.
6. Add the garlic and ginger, cook for 1 minute before adding the kale and cabbage. Cook for 2-3 minutes, stirring frequently, until the kale and cabbage begin to wilt. Add the carrot and soy sauce and cook for another 2 minutes.

7. Serve the veggies over the cooked noodles and top with the tofu. Eat immediately.

14. Syn Free Cheesy Oven Baked Meatball Subs

Total Time: 30 Min

Ingredients

- 3x Large Tomatoes (roughly chopped)
- Half a Pack Cherry Tomatoes (halved)
- 2tbsp Tomato Puree
- 150mls Boiling Chicken Stock (or veg stock)
- Pack of Muscle Foods Giant British Meatballs (cut into quarters)
- 3tbsp Mixed Herbs
- 70g Grated Mozzarella (2 person's HexA choice, some varieties allow 40g per person)
- 2x Crusty Wholemeal Rolls (60g each, remove bread from the middle if too heavy - cut in half)
- Salt & Pepper (to taste)

- Fry Light

Directions

1. Preheat your grill to 200 degrees.

2. In a frying pan, fry your quartered meatballs until cooked through.

3. Meanwhile, spray a medium sauce pan over a high heat with Fry Light and add your chopped tomatoes and cherry tomatoes. Fry until they begin to break down.

4. Add the stock, two tablespoons of the herbs and some salt and pepper to taste and reduce the heat. Simmer for 5-10 minutes.

5. Add the tomato puree and simmer until the sauce has thickened. Mix in your meatballs.

6. While your sauce is thickening, spray a baking tray with Fry Light and then place your halved rolls in it crust side down. Spray with a bit of Fry Light and pop under the grill for two minutes to toast.

7. When toasted, remove from the oven and evenly spoon the meatballs and sauce onto the rolls.

8. Sprinkle over your cheese, and the rest of the herbs, and place back under the grill to broil.

9. Once the cheese has melted, take out of the oven and serve immediately!

15. Chicken Stir-Fry

Total: 30 min

Prep: 10 min

Cook: 20 min

Yield: 4 servings

Ingredients

- 2 tablespoons dark sesame oil, divided
- 2 garlic cloves, finely minced
- 2 pounds chicken breasts, skinless and boneless
- 1 head broccoli, stems removed
- 1 dozen mushrooms, sliced
- 3 carrots, peeled and julienned
- 1/4 pound green beans, diced
- 1 head bok choy, chopped
- 2 to 3 tablespoons teriyaki sauce

Directions

1. Heat 1 tablespoon oil in a saute pan over medium heat. Add garlic and stir. Place the chicken in the

pan and brown 4 minutes on each side. Remove from pan, slice into strips, set aside.

2. Heat remaining tablespoon of oil in a wok over high heat. Add the vegetables and teriyaki sauce. Stir-fry quickly until the vegetables begin to soften. Add the chicken strips, combine well and continue to cook for 2 to 3 minutes. Serve immediately.

16. Stuffed Sweet Potatoes with Curry Chickpeas

Prep Time: 10 mins

Cook Time: 20 mins

Total Time: 30 mins

Servings: 3 -4

Ingredients

- ¼ - ½ cup canola oil
- 2 -3 tablespoon curry powder
- 1 large onion diced
- 2 teaspoons minced garlic
- teaspoon ground allspice
- teaspoon ground nutmeg spice
- 1½ teaspoon smoked paprika
- 2 teaspoons fresh or dried thyme
- teaspoon cumin spice
- teaspoon white pepper.
- 2 cans of chickpeas drained
- 1-2 cups of cubed potatoes
- ½ - tablespoon bouillon chicken powder optional

- 1 cup or more broth or water
- 1 cup coconut milk replace with broth or water
- ½-1 teaspoon cayenne pepper optional
- 2 green onions chopped
- 1-2 cups fresh leaf spinach
- 2 tablespoons or more chopped parsley
- Salt to taste

Directions

1. Heat up large sauce-pan with oil, and add onions, garlic, thyme, cumin spice, all spice, smoked paprika, nutmeg and curry powder, stir occasionally for about 2-3 minutes until onions is translucent.
2. Then add potatoes, stir and sauté for about 2-3 more minutes. Add coconut milk /stock / water if necessary to prevent any burns
3. Next add chickpeas, green onion and broth. Bring to a boil and let it simmer until sauce thickens, it might take about 18 minutes.

4. Lastly throw in some spinach ,parsley, adjust for salt, pepper and stew consistency. Stir for about a minute until spinach is wilted .Serve warm

5. While curry is simmering. Cook sweet potatoes in your microwave: Prick the potatoes all over with a fork. Microwave on high for 8 to 10 minutes or until sweet potatoes is tender, turning the potatoes once. Clean and dry the sweet potatoes, poke holes into the sweet potatoes, place in the microwave and cook for about 4 minutes. Remove , let cook for a couple of minutes Slice open the sweet potatoes and stuff! If your sweet potatoes are large, cut them in half.

17. Green Juice in a Blender

Prep: 10 Minutes

Yield: 4 Servings

Ingredients

- 1 1/2 cups water
- 2 cups kale
- 2 green apples, cored
- 1/2 cup parsley leaves
- 1 medium cucumber, quartered
- 2 celery stalks, roughly chopped
- 1 (1-inch) piece of ginger, peeled
- 2 Tablespoons lemon juice

Equipment:

- blender; fine mesh sieve (optional)

Directions

1. Add all of the ingredients into the blender jug in the order in which they are listed. Blend the ingredients on the highest level setting, such as

"liquefy," until the juice is well-blended. (It will be the consistency of a smoothie.)

2. If you want to enjoy the pulp with your juice, pour the mixture into glasses and serve. If you prefer a thinner consistency, pour the mixture through a fine mesh sieve, and using a spatula, press the pulp into the sieve to extract as much liquid as possible. Pour the strained juice into glasses and serve.

18. Miso Ramen Soup with Buckwheat Noodles

Preparation Time: Over 2 Hours

Cooking Time: Less Than 10 Mins

Serves: 4

Ingredients

For the bone broth

- 1.5kg beef bones, chicken carcasses, lamb bones (usually free from the butchers) or use the saved bones from a roast

- splash of apple cider vinegar or fresh lemon juice (optional – this can help to extract the minerals from the meat bones)
- 1 handful of any onions, leeks, carrots or celery ends
- 1 tbsp black peppercorns
- 2 bay leaves

For the noodles and vegetables

- 350g/12oz buckwheat noodles
- 1 tbsp sesame oil or extra virgin olive oil
- 4 heads pak choi, trimmed and thinly sliced
- 200g/7oz mixed mushrooms, sliced
- 1 carrot, julienned
- ½ red cabbage, stalk removed, leaves shredded
- 5cm/2in piece fresh root ginger, peeled, grated
- 6 spring onions, trimmed, finely sliced on the diagonal
- 4 tbsp lime juice
- 2 tbsp miso paste, preferably unpasteurised
- 1-2 tsp tamari or salt, to taste

- large handful chopped fresh coriander, to serve

Directions

1. Put all of the ingredients for the bone broth in a large lidded pot and cover with cold water. The water level should cover the bones by 5cm/2in while still leaving room at the top of the pan. Cover and bring to the boil. Reduce the heat and simmer for at least 6 hours for chicken and 12 for beef or lamb, skimming off any foam that rises to the top. Strain the liquid and return to the pot, set aside.

2. Cook the buckwheat noodles according to the packet instructions, using plenty of water. During the first minute of cooking, use two forks to stir and separate the noodles.

3. Drain the cooked noodles and rinse under cold running water for 15-20 seconds to stop them cooking any further. Set aside to drain, then drizzle over a little sesame oil and mix through to prevent the noodles from sticking to each other.

4. Divide the pak choy, mushrooms, carrot and red cabbage equally among four serving bowls.

5. Gently heat the bone broth and stir in the grated ginger, spring onions, lime juice, miso paste and tamari.

6. Pour the hot broth over the vegetables, sprinkle the coriander on top and serve.

19. Good-for-you Granola

Prep: 10 Mins

Cook: 25 Mins

Makes 15 Servings

Ingredients

- 2 tbsp vegetable oil
- 125ml maple syrup
- 2 tbsp honey
- 1 tsp vanilla extract
- 300g rolled oats
- 50g sunflower seed
- 4 tbsp sesame seeds
- 50g pumpkin seeds
- 100g flaked almond
- 100g dried berries (find them in the baking aisle)

- 50g coconut

- flakes or desiccated coconut

Directions

1. Heat oven to 150C/fan 130C/gas 2. Mix the oil, maple syrup, honey and vanilla in a large bowl. Tip in all the remaining ingredients, except the dried fruit and coconut, and mix well.

2. Tip the granola onto two baking sheets and spread evenly. Bake for 15 mins, then mix in the coconut and dried fruit, and bake for 10-15 mins more. Remove and scrape onto a flat tray to cool. Serve with cold milk or yogurt. The granola can be stored in an airtight container for up to a month.

20. Salmon Salad

Prep Time: 20 minutes

Cook Time: 15 minutes

Total Time: 35 minutes

Servings: 4

Ingredients

For the salad

- 1 pound salmon fillets 3-4 ounces each
- 1 teaspoon dried italian seasoning
- salt and pepper to taste
- 2 teaspoons olive oil
- 4 cups romaine lettuce chopped
- 1 cup cherry tomatoes halved
- 1 cup cucumber quartered and sliced
- 1/2 cup kalamata olives halved
- 1/4 cup red onion thinly sliced
- 1/3 cup feta cheese crumbled
- 1/4 cup fresh dill minced
- 1/2 cup green bell pepper chopped
- 1 avocado peeled, pitted and sliced

For the dressing

- 1/4 cup olive oil
- 1 teaspoon Dijon mustard
- 2 tablespoons red wine vinegar
- 1 tablespoon lemon juice
- 1/4 teaspoon garlic powder
- 1/4 teaspoon onion powder
- 1/2 teaspoon dried oregano
- salt and pepper to taste

Directions

1. Season the salmon fillets with the Italian seasoning, salt and pepper.
2. Heat the 2 teaspoons olive oil in a large pan over high heat.
3. Add the salmon and cook for 4-6 minutes per side or until browned and cooked through.
4. While the salmon is cooking, place the lettuce, tomato, cucumber, olives, red onion, feta, dill and bell pepper in a large bowl. Toss gently to combine. Arrange the avocado over the top.

5. In a small bowl, whisk together all the ingredients for the dressing.

6. Let the salmon cool for 5-7 minutes. Place the salmon fillets over the lettuce mixture. Drizzle the dressing over the salad, then serve.

21. Spanish stuffed marrow

Prep: 20 Mins

Cook: 1 Hr

Serves: 6

Ingredients

- 1 marrow
- 1 tbsp olive oil
- 1 onion, diced
- 2 garlic cloves, crushed
- 100g chorizo, chopped
- 1 tsp smoked paprika
- ½ tsp cayenne pepper
- ½ tsp each dried oregano and dried thyme
- 2 x 400g cans chopped tomatoes
- 140g roasted red pepper from a jar, sliced
- handful parsley, chopped
- 85g fresh breadcrumb
- 100g manchego, grated

Directions

1. Heat oven to 200C/180C fan/gas 6. Cut the marrow in half lengthways and scoop out the middle. Put the halves, cut-side up, in a large roasting tin and season.

2. Heat the oil in a saucepan, add the onion and sweat on a low heat for 10 mins until soft. Add the garlic, chorizo, spices and dried herbs. Cook for a few mins, then add the tomatoes and peppers. Turn down to a low simmer and cook for 10 mins, then stir through the parsley.

3. Spoon the tomato mixture into the marrow halves, cover with foil and bake for 30 mins. Sprinkle over the breadcrumbs and Manchego, and return to the oven for 10 mins until the crumbs are golden and crisp, and the marrow is tender.

22. Griddled Courgette & Seafood Lasagne

Prep: 10 Mins

Cook: 40 Mins

Serves: 4

Ingredients

- 1 tsp oil
- 4 courgettes, sliced lengthways
- 1 red chilli, deseeded and finely chopped
- ½ x 680ml jar passata with onion and garlic
- 400g bag seafood mix, defrosted if frozen
- 4 fresh lasagne sheets, halved
- 3 tbsp grated parmesan
- 3 tbsp dried breadcrumbs
- 350g green bean, to serve

Directions

1. Heat a griddle and brush a little oil on the courgettes. Cook in batches until lightly charred. Season and scatter on the chilli, then set aside.

2. Heat oven to 200C/180C fan/gas 6. Pour a little passata in a medium-sized ovenproof dish. Place half the seafood over it, then season and top with a third of the courgettes.

3. Top with 2 sheets of pasta, then more tomato sauce, seafood, courgettes, another layer of pasta, more tomato sauce and finish with the rest of the courgettes. Mix the Parmesan and breadcrumbs, then scatter on top and cook for 25-30 mins until golden. Steam or boil the green beans and serve with the lasagne.

23. Creamy Pumpkin & Lentil Soup

Prep: 15 Mins

Cook: 35 Mins

Serves: 4

Ingredients

- 1 tbsp olive oil, plus 1 tsp
- 2 onions, chopped
- 2 garlic cloves, chopped
- approx 800g chopped pumpkin flesh, plus the seeds
- 100g split red lentil
- ½ small pack thyme, leaves picked, plus extra to serve
- 1l hot vegetable stock
- pinch of salt and sugar
- 50g crème fraîche, plus extra to serve

Directions

1. Heat the oil in a large pan. Fry the onions until softened and starting to turn golden. Stir in the

garlic, pumpkin flesh, lentils and thyme, then pour in the hot stock. Season, cover and simmer for 20-25 mins until the lentils and vegetables are tender.

2. Meanwhile, wash the pumpkin seeds. Remove any flesh still clinging to them, then dry them with kitchen paper. Heat the 1 tsp oil in a non-stick pan and fry the seeds until they start to jump and pop. Stir frequently, but cover the pan in between to keep them in it. When the seeds look nutty and toasted, add a sprinkling of salt and a pinch of sugar, and stir well.

3. Whizz the cooked pumpkin mixture with a hand blender or in a food processor until smooth, then add the crème fraîche and whizz again. Taste for seasoning.

4. Serve with a spoonful of crème fraîche, a few thyme leaves and the toasted seeds scattered on top.

24. Asian Chicken Salad

Prep: 10 Mins

Cook: 10 Mins

Serves: 2

Ingredients

- 1 boneless, skinless chicken breast
- 1 tbsp fish sauce
- zest and juice ½ lime (about 1 tbsp)
- 1 tsp caster sugar
- 100g bag mixed salad leaves
- large handful coriander, roughly chopped
- ¼ red onion, thinly sliced
- ½ chilli, deseeded and thinly sliced
- ¼ cucumber, halved lengthways, sliced

Directions

1. Cover the chicken with cold water, bring to the boil, then cook for 10 mins. Remove from the pan and tear into shreds. Stir together the fish sauce, lime zest, juice and sugar until sugar dissolves.

2. Place the leaves and coriander in a container, then
   top with the chicken, onion, chilli and cucumber.
   Place the dressing in a separate container and toss
   through the salad when ready to eat.

25. Mushroom, Spinach & Potato Pie

Prep: 15 Mins

Cook: 45 Mins

Serves: 4

Ingredients

- 400g baby spinach
- 1 tbsp olive oil
- 500g mushroom, such as chestnut, shiitake and
  button
- 2 garlic cloves, crushed
- 250ml vegetable stock (made from half a low
  sodium vegetable stock cube)
- 300g cooked new potatoes, cut into bite-sized
  pieces
- 1 tbsp grain mustard
- 1 tsp freshly grated nutmeg

- 2 heaped tbsp light crème fraîche
- 3 sheets filo pastry
- 300g each green beans and broccoli, steamed

Directions

1. Heat oven to 200C/180C fan/gas 6. Wilt spinach in a colander by pouring a kettleful of hot water over it.

2. Heat half the oil in a large non-stick pan and fry mushrooms on a high heat until golden. Add garlic and cook for 1 min, then tip in stock, mustard, nutmeg and potatoes. Bubble for a few mins until reduced. Season, then remove from the heat; add crème fraîche and spinach. Pour into a pie dish and allow to cool for a few mins.

3. Brush filo with remaining oil, quarter sheets then loosely scrunch up and lay on top of pie filling. Bake for 20-25 mins until golden. Serve with vegetables.

26. Ricotta, Tomato & Spinach Frittata

Prep: 10 Mins

Cook: 35 Mins

Serves: 4

Ingredients

- 1 tbsp olive oil
- 1 large onion, finely sliced
- 300g cherry tomatoes
- 100g spinach leaves
- small handful basil leaves
- 100g ricotta
- 6 eggs, beaten
- salad, to serve

Directions

1. Heat oven to 200C/180C fan/gas 6. Heat oil in a large non-stick frying pan and cook the onion for 5-6 mins until softened and lightly golden. Add the tomatoes and toss for 1 min to soften.

2. Remove from the heat, add the spinach leaves and basil, and toss together to wilt a little. Transfer all the ingredients to a greased 30cm x 20cm rectangular baking tin. Take small scoops of the ricotta and dot over the vegetables.

3. Season the eggs and beat well, then pour over the vegetables and cheese. Cook in the oven for 20-25 mins until pale golden and set. Serve with salad.

27. Turkish One-pan Eggs & Peppers (Menemen)

Prep: 10 Mins

Cook: 25 Mins

Serves: 4

Ingredients

- 2 tbsp olive oil
- 2 onions, sliced
- 1 red or green pepper, halved deseeded and sliced
- 1-2 red chillies, deseeded and sliced
- 400g can chopped tomatoes
- 1-2 tsp caster sugar

- 4 eggs
- small bunch parsley, roughly chopped
- 6 tbsp thick, creamy yogurt
- 2 garlic cloves, crushed

Directions

1. Heat the oil in a heavy-based frying pan. Stir in the onions, pepper and chillies. Cook until they begin to soften. Add the tomatoes and sugar, mixing well. Cook until the liquid has reduced, season.

2. Using a wooden spoon, create 4 pockets in the tomato mixture and crack the eggs into them. Cover the pan and cook the eggs over a low heat until just set.

3. Beat the yogurt with the garlic and season. Sprinkle the menemen with parsley and serve from the frying pan with a dollop of the garlic-flavoured yogurt.

28. Teriyaki Salmon Parcels

Prep: 15 Mins

Cook: 20 Mins

Serves: 4

Ingredients

- 2 tbsp low-salt soy sauce
- 1 tbsp clear honey
- 1 garlic clove, finely chopped
- 1 tbsp mirin (optional)
- a little sunflower oil
- 300g Tenderstem broccoli
- 4 x 100g salmon fillets
- 1 small piece of ginger, cut into matchsticks
- a little sesame oil (optional)
- sliced spring onions, toasted sesame seeds and cooked rice, to serve

Directions

1. KIDS: The writing in bold is for you. ADULTS: The rest is for you. Make the sauce and marinade. In a small bowl, whisk together the soy, honey, garlic and mirin and set aside.

2. Cut out some squares of foil. Using scissors, cut out 4 squares of foil, each about 30cm square. Brush each piece of foil with a little oil and bring the edges of the foil up a little.

3. Fill your parcels. Place a couple of broccoli stems on each one, then sit a salmon fillet on top and scatter over the ginger.

4. Spoon over the sauce. Spoon the sauce over each salmon fillet and drizzle with a little sesame oil, if you like.

5. Close the parcels. Fold over the edges of the foil together to seal and place the parcels on a baking sheet. Can be prepared up to 1 day ahead.

6. Cook the parcels. Heat oven to 200C/180C fan/gas 6. Get your child to place the parcels in the oven for 15-20 mins, but ensure an adult removes them, then leave to stand for a few mins. Serve each

parcel on a plate and let each person open it themselves. Serve with spring onions and sesame seeds for scattering over, and some rice on the side.

29. Broccoli and Kale Green Soup

Prep: 15 Mins

Cook: 20 Mins

Serves: 2

Ingredients

- 500ml stock, made by mixing 1 tbsp bouillon powder and boiling water in a jug
- 1 tbsp sunflower oil
- 2 garlic cloves, sliced
- thumb-sized piece ginger, sliced
- ½ tsp ground coriander
- 3cm/1in piece fresh turmeric root, peeled and grated, or ½ tsp ground turmeric
- pinch of pink Himalayan salt
- 200g courgettes, roughly sliced
- 85g broccoli

- 100g kale, chopped

- 1 lime, zested and juiced

- small pack parsley, roughly chopped, reserving a few whole leaves to serve

Directions

1. Put the oil in a deep pan, add the garlic, ginger, coriander, turmeric and salt, fry on a medium heat for 2 mins, then add 3 tbsp water to give a bit more moisture to the spices.

2. Add the courgettes, making sure you mix well to coat the slices in all the spices, and continue cooking for 3 mins. Add 400ml stock and leave to simmer for 3 mins.

3. Add the broccoli, kale and lime juice with the rest of the stock. Leave to cook again for another 3-4 mins until all the vegetables are soft.

4. Take off the heat and add the chopped parsley. Pour everything into a blender and blend on high speed until smooth. It will be a beautiful green with bits of dark speckled through (which is the kale). Garnish with lime zest and parsley.

30. Chickpea, Tomato & Spinach Curry

Prep: 15 Mins

Cook: 40 Mins

Serves: 6

Ingredients

- 1 onion, chopped
- 2 garlic cloves, chopped
- 3cm/1¼ in piece ginger, grated
- 6 ripe tomatoes
- ½ tbsp oil
- 1 tsp ground cumin
- 2 tsp ground coriander
- 1 tsp turmeric
- pinch chilli flakes
- 1 tsp yeast extract (we used Marmite)
- 4 tbsp red lentils
- 6 tbsp coconut cream
- 1 head of broccoli, broken into small florets
- 400g can chickpeas, drained
- 100g bag baby spinach leaves

- 1 lemon, halved

- 1 tbsp toasted sesame seed

- 1 tbsp chopped cashew, to mix with the sesame seeds

Directions

1. Put the onion, garlic, ginger and tomatoes in a food processor or blender and whizz to a purée.

2. Heat oil in a large pan. Add the spices, fry for a few secs and add purée and yeast extract. Bubble together for 2 mins, then add lentils and coconut cream. Cook until lentils are tender, then add the broccoli and cook for 4 mins. Stir in chickpeas and spinach, squeeze over lemon and swirl through sesame and cashew mixture. Serve with brown rice, if you like.

31. Vanilla Chai Breakfast Smoothie

Serves: 1

- ¼ cup unsweetened almond milk
- ¼ cup chai tea (brewed from a teabag and chilled)
- ½ scoop plant-based vanilla protein powder
- ½ frozen banana
- ½ tsp ground cinnamon
- 2 tbsp oats
- water to blend (optional)

32. Peanut Butter Cup

Serves: 1

- ½ cup unsweetened almond milk
- 1 scoop vanilla or chocolate plant-based protein powder
- 1 tbsp unsweetened cocoa powder
- ½ frozen banana
- ½ tbsp natural unsalted peanut butter
- water to blend (optional)

33. Fresh Blueberry

Serves: 1

- ½ cup unsweetened almond milk
- 1 scoop vanilla plant-based protein powder
- ½ cup frozen blueberries
- ½ tbsp natural unsalted almond butter
- water to blend (optional)

34. Green Monster

- ¼ cup no-sugar-added apple juice
- ¼ cup water
- ½ scoop plant-based vanilla protein powder
- ½ Bosc pear, chopped
- ½ cup baby spinach, loosely packed
- ½ frozen banana
- ¼ ripe avocado